Non Gallbladder Super Diet Cookbook Dishes

Simple Delicious Wholesome Flavourful Recipes To Aid Digestion Reduce Inflammatory After Gallbladder Removal

Nancy V. Goss

Copyright © by Nancy V. Goss 2024. All rights reserved.
Before this document is duplicated or reproduced in any manner, the publisher's consent must be gained. Therefore, the contents within can neither be stored electronically, transferred, nor kept in a database. Neither in Part nor full can the document be copied, scanned, faxed, or retained without approval from the publisher or creator.

Table Of Contents

INTRODUCTION
Understanding gallbladder health and diet

Chapter 1
Breakfast Dishes
Whole wheat toast with avocado and tomato
Broccoli and feta frittata

Chapter 2
Soups and Salads
Arugula and pear salad with walnuts
Chicken and brown rice soup

Chapter 3
Main Dishes
Turkey meatballs with whole-grain pasta
Baked cod with tomatoes and capers

Chapter 4
Sides and Snacks
Hummus with carrots and celery sticks
Cucumber and avocado roll-ups

Chapter 5
Appetizer
Homemade Ravioli with Ricotta and Spinach Filling
Tuna Tartare with Caper Dressing

Chapter 6
Dessert
Dark chocolate dipped strawberries with sauce
Lemon Poppyseed Muffins

CONCLUSION

INTRODUCTION

Rita, a resilient woman in her early 50s, had been struggling with her health ever since her gallbladder was removed three years ago. She experienced bloating, pain, and discomfort after eating, despite following her doctor's recommendations. One day, while browsing online, Rita stumbled upon a book titled "Non-Gallbladder Super Diet Cookbook Dishes." Intrigued, she decided to give it a try and purchased the book.

As she delved into the cookbook, Rita discovered a wealth of information on how to adapt her diet to her new reality. The book provided invaluable insights into the importance of low-fat meals, and it offered an array of delicious, easy-to-follow recipes. Eager to regain control of her health, Rita set out to incorporate these new dishes into her daily life.

Almost instantly, Rita noticed significant improvements in her digestion, energy levels, and overall well being. As she continued experimenting with the cookbook's recipes, her symptoms gradually subsided, and she began to feel like her old self again.

With gratitude for the serendipitous discovery of the "Non-Gallbladder Super Diet Cookbook Dishes," Rita continued to spread hope, wisdom, and the joy of delicious food to countless people, reminding everyone that even in the face of adversity, there is always an opportunity for growth and connection.

Understanding gallbladder health and diet

Understanding gallbladder health and diet is crucial for maintaining optimal digestive function and overall wellbeing. The gallbladder is a small, pear-shaped organ located beneath the liver that stores and concentrates bile, a digestive fluid produced by the liver. Bile helps break down fats in the small intestine, enabling the absorption of fat-soluble vitamins and nutrients.

Several factors can affect gallbladder health, including:

1. Diet: A diet high in unhealthy fats, refined carbohydrates, and low in fiber may increase the risk of gallbladder problems.

2. Obesity: Excess body weight is associated with a higher risk of gallbladder issues, such as gallstones.

3. Genetics: A family history of gallbladder problems may predispose an individual to develop similar issues.

4. Age: The risk of gallbladder problems increases with age.

A gallbladder-friendly diet should focus on the following principles:

1. Low in unhealthy fats: Limit saturated fats, found in fatty meats and full-fat dairy products, and trans fats, found in processed foods. Instead, choose healthier fats, like omega-3 fatty acids in fish and monounsaturated fats in avocados and nuts.

2. High in fiber: Consume plenty of fruits, vegetables, and whole grains to ensure adequate fiber intake, which aids in digestion and maintains regular bowel movements.

3. Lean protein: Opt for lean protein sources, such as poultry, fish, tofu, and legumes, to support muscle health without overburdening the gallbladder.

4. Hydration: Drink plenty of water throughout the day to support healthy bile production and maintain overall digestive function.

5. Healthy weight management: Achieving and maintaining a healthy weight can reduce the risk of gallbladder issues.

In cases where the gallbladder is removed due to chronic issues, such as gallstones or inflammation, the body can still digest food.

However, a low-fat diet is often recommended to help ease the digestive process and minimize post-surgery discomfort. Working with a healthcare professional or registered dietitian can ensure a tailored approach to dietary management for optimal gallbladder health.

Chapter 1

Breakfast Dishes

Whole wheat toast with avocado and tomato
Prep Time: 10 minutes
Ingredients:
2 slices whole wheat bread
1/2 ripe avocado
1 small tomato, sliced
Salt and pepper, to taste
1/2 teaspoon lemon juice (optional)
Fresh herbs (cilantro or parsley), chopped (optional)
Red pepper flakes (optional)

Instructions:
1. Toast the whole wheat bread slices in a toaster until they reach your desired level of crispiness.
2. While the bread is toasting, prepare the avocado mash. Slice the avocado also in half and take away the pit. Scoop out the flesh well into a small bowl.
3. Mash the avocado using a fork or a potato masher. Add salt and pepper to taste. For extra flavor, you can also add a squeeze of lemon juice and a pinch of red pepper flakes.
4. Spread the mashed avocado evenly on the toasted bread slices very well.

5. Layer the sliced tomatoes on top of the avocado toast.
6. If desired, sprinkle fresh herbs (such as cilantro or parsley) on top of the tomatoes.
7. Season with additional salt and pepper very well, if need
8. Serve immediately and enjoy your delicious and nutritious whole wheat toast with avocado and tomato.

Broccoli and feta frittata

Prep Time: 10 minutes
Cook Time: 20-25 minutes
Ingredients:
6 large eggs
1/2 cup milk
Salt and pepper, to taste
2 cups broccoli florets, chopped
1/2 cup feta cheese, crumbled
1/4 cup onion, diced
2 cloves garlic, minced
2 tablespoons olive oil

Instructions:
1. Preheat the oven to 375°F (190°C) and prepare a 9-inch pie dish or oven-safe skillet by greasing it with cooking spray or a bit of oil.
2. In a large bowl, whisk the eggs together with milk, salt, and pepper until well combined.
3. Heat the olive oil in a non-stick skillet over a small heat. Add the diced onion and minced garlic and sauté for two-three minutes until softened and fragrant.
4. Add the chopped broccoli florets to the skillet and cook for another 5-6 minutes, stirring occasionally, until they become bright green and slightly tender. Season with salt and pepper to taste very well.

5. Pour the cooked broccoli mixture into the prepared pie dish or skillet, spreading it evenly.

Pour the egg mixture over the broccoli mixture. Sprinkle the crumbled feta cheese on top also.

6. Bake a frittata in the preheated oven for 20-25 minutes or until the eggs are set, and the top is golden brown.

7. Remove the frittata from the oven and let it cool for a few minutes before slicing.

8. Serve your Broccoli and Feta Frittata warm or at room temperature, alongside a fresh green salad or whole-grain toast for a well-rounded meal. This recipe makes four- six servings, depending on portion size.

Chapter 2

Soups and Salads

Arugula and pear salad with walnuts

Prep Time: 15 minutes
Ingredients:
6 cups baby arugula
2 ripe pears, cored and thinly sliced
1/2 cup walnut halves, toasted and roughly chopped
Half cup crumbled goat cheese or blue cheese
1/4 cup dried cranberries (optional)

Lemon Vinaigrette:
1/4 cup extra-virgin olive oil
2 tablespoons fresh lemon juice
1 teaspoon honey
1/2 teaspoon Dijon mustard
Salt and freshly ground black pepper, to taste

Instructions:
2. In a small bowl or jar, whisk together the olive oil, lemon juice, honey, Dijon mustard, salt, and pepper to make the lemon vinaigrette.
2. In a large mixing bowl, combine the baby arugula, sliced pears, toasted walnuts, crumbled cheese, and dried cranberries (if using).

3. Drizzle the lemon vinaigrette over the salad ingredients and gently toss to coat everything evenly.

Serve the Arugula and Pear Salad with Walnuts immediately, as the arugula will begin to wilt once dressed.

Chicken and brown rice soup

Prep Time: 15 minutes
Cook Time: 50-55 minutes
Ingredients:
1 tablespoon olive oil
One lb boneless, skinless chicken breasts or thighs
1 medium onion, diced
3 medium carrots, sliced
3 celery stalks, sliced
2 garlic cloves, minced
1 teaspoon dried thyme
1 teaspoon dried oregano
6 cups low-sodium chicken broth
1 cup uncooked brown rice
Salt and pepper, to taste
Fresh parsley, chopped (optional)
Lemon wedges (optional)

Instructions:
1. Heat the olive oil in a large pot or Dutch oven over a small heat.
2. Add the chicken and cook until lightly browned on all sides, about 5-6 minutes.
3. Remove the chicken from the pot and set it aside to rest.
4. In the same pot, sauté the onions, carrots, and celery until they soften, approximately 5-6 minutes.

5. Add the minced garlic, dried thyme, and dried oregano, and cook for another minute until fragrant.

6. Pour in the chicken broth, and add the brown rice to the pot. Stir well.

7. Cut the rested chicken into bite-sized pieces or shred it with a fork, then return it to the pot.

8. Bring the soup to a boil, then reduce the heat to low and let it simmer for 35-40 minutes, or until the brown rice is cooked and tender.

9. Taste the soup and season with salt and pepper as needed.

Serve the warm Chicken and Brown Rice Soup with a sprinkle of fresh parsley and a lemon wedge on the side for added flavor

Chapter 3

Main Dishes

Turkey meatballs with whole-grain pasta

Prep Time: 15 minutes
Cook Time: 25-30 minutes
Ingredients:
For the turkey meatballs:
1 lb. ground turkey (preferably lean or extra-lean)
1/2 cup whole-grain breadcrumbs
1/4 cup grated Parmesan cheese
1/4 cup finely chopped onion
1/4 cup chopped fresh parsley
1 large egg, beaten
1 teaspoon Italian seasoning
1/2 teaspoon garlic powder
Salt and pepper, to taste

For the pasta and sauce:
12 oz. whole-grain pasta (like spaghetti)
24 oz. marinara or tomato sauce
Optional: fresh basil leaves and additional Parmesan cheese for serving

Instructions:
1. Preheat the oven to Four hundred°F (200°C)
2. In a large mixing bowl, combine the ground turkey, breadcrumbs, Parmesan cheese, chopped onion, parsley, beaten egg, Italian seasoning, garlic powder, salt, and pepper. Mix/stir well using your hands or a wooden spoon.
3. Form the mixture into golf-ball-sized meatballs and place them on the prepared baking sheet.
4. Bake the meatballs in the preheated oven for 20-25 minutes or until they're fully cooked and golden brown.
5. While the meatballs are baking, cook the whole-grain pasta according to the package instructions. Drain and set aside.
6. In a large saucepan, heat the marinara or tomato sauce over medium heat.
7. Once the meatballs are cooked, add them to the saucepan with the sauce and simmer for 5 minutes, stirring occasionally.
8. Serve the turkey meatballs and sauce over the cooked whole-grain pasta, garnished with fresh basil leaves and additional Parmesan cheese, if desired.

Baked cod with tomatoes and capers

Prep Time: 10 minutes
Cook Time: 20-25 minutes
Ingredients:
4 cod fillets (about 6 oz each)
2 tablespoons olive oil
1 pint cherry tomatoes, halved
2 tablespoons capers, drained
2 garlic cloves, minced
1/2 teaspoon dried thyme
Salt and pepper, to taste
Fresh parsley, chopped (optional)

Instructions:
1. Preheat the oven to 400°F (200°C).
2. In a large oven-safe skillet or baking dish, arrange the cod fillets in a single layer.
3. Drizzle the olive oil over the fillets and season them with salt and pepper.
4. Scatter the halved cherry tomatoes and capers around the fillets, ensuring even distribution.
5. Sprinkle the minced garlic and dried thyme over the fish and vegetables.
6. Bake the cod in the preheated oven for 20-25 minutes, or until the fish flakes easily with a fork.
7. Garnish the baked cod with chopped fresh parsley, if desired.Serve the Baked Cod with Tomatoes and Capers immediately, paired with your favorite side dish, such as whole-grain rice, quinoa, or roasted vegetables.

Chapter 4

Sides and Snacks

Hummus with carrots and celery sticks

Prep Time: 10 minutes
Ingredients:
For the hummus:
One (fifteen oz.) can chickpeas, drained and liquid reserved
1/4 cup tahini
1/4 cup lemon juice
1 garlic clove, minced
1/2 teaspoon ground cumin
Salt and pepper, to taste
2-4 tablespoons chickpea liquid or water
For serving:
Carrots, peeled and cut into sticks
Celery stalks, cut into sticks

Instructions:
2. In a food processor or blender, combine the drained chickpeas, tahini, lemon juice, minced garlic, ground cumin, salt, and pepper.

2. Blend the ingredients until they form a thick paste, stopping the processor occasionally to scrape down the sides as needed.
3. With the motor running, slowly add 2 tablespoons of the reserved chickpea liquid or water to the mixture until you reach your desired consistency. For a creamier hummus, add more liquid, 1 tablespoon at a time.
4. Taste the hummus and adjust the seasonings as needed.
5. Serve the hummus with the carrot and celery sticks for a healthy, crunchy snack or appetizer.

This simple Hummus with Carrots and Celery Sticks recipe is perfect for sharing with friends and family or enjoying as a nutritious, satisfying snack.

Cucumber and avocado roll-ups

Prep Time: 15 minutes

Ingredients:
1 large cucumber, sliced into thin strips with a vegetable peeler or mandoline
1 ripe avocado, mashed
1/4 cup cream cheese, softened
1 tablespoon lime juice
1/4 teaspoon garlic powder
Salt and pepper, to taste
Fresh herbs (like cilantro or parsley),
Toothpicks for securing roll-ups

Instructions:
1. In a small mixing bowl, combine the mashed avocado, softened cream cheese, lime juice, garlic powder, salt, and pepper. Stir well to blend the ingredients evenly.
2. Lay out the thin cucumber strips on a clean work surface.
3. Spread a thin layer of the avocado mixture onto each cucumber strip, leaving a small border around the edges.
4. If desired, sprinkle chopped fresh herbs over the avocado mixture.
5. Carefully roll up each cucumber strip, starting at one end and rolling tightly toward the other end.

6. Secure the cucumber roll-ups with a toothpick to keep them in place.

Serve the Cucumber and Avocado Roll-Ups chilled or at room temperature as a healthy and refreshing snack, appetizer, or addition to a meal.

Chapter 5

Appetizer

Homemade Ravioli with Ricotta and Spinach Filling

Ingredients:
- 2 cups all-purpose flour
- 2 large eggs
- 1/2 teaspoon salt
- 1 tablespoon olive oil
- 1 cup ricotta cheese
- 1 cup chopped spinach
- 1/4 cup grated Parmesan cheese
- Salt and pepper to taste
- Your favorite pasta sauce, for serving

Instructions:
1. In a medium mixing bowl, combine the flour and salt. Make a well in the center and crack the eggs well into it. Add the olive oil and mix until a dough forms.
2. Knead the dough on a floured surface for about 5 minutes, until smooth and elastic. Cover with a damp cloth and let it rest for thirty minutes.
3. In a separate bowl, mix together the ricotta cheese, chopped spinach, Parmesan cheese, salt, and pepper.

4. Roll out the dough on a floured surface until about 1/8 inch thick. Cut into squares or circles, depending on your portion size.

5. Place a spoonful of the ricotta and spinach mixture onto half of the dough pieces. Brush the edges with water and top with another piece of dough. Press the edges together to seal.

6. Bring a large pot of salted water to heat. Cook the ravioli for about 4-5 minutes, or until they float to the surface.

7. Serve the ravioli with your favorite pasta sauce and enjoy!

Prep time: 1 hour 15 minutes

Tuna Tartare with Caper Dressing

Ingredients:
- 1 lb sushi-grade tuna, diced
- 2 tbsp capers, drained and chopped
- 2 tbsp red onion, finely chopped
- 2 tbsp fresh parsley, chopped
- 1 tbsp Dijon mustard
- 2 tbsp extra virgin olive oil
- 1 tbsp lemon juice
- Salt and pepper, to taste
- Crostini or crackers, for serving

Instructions:
1. In a mixing bowl, combine the diced tuna, capers, red onion, and parsley.
2. In a small bowl, whisk together the Dijon mustard, olive oil, lemon juice, salt, and pepper.
3. Pour the dressing over the tuna mixture and toss until well combined.
4. Cover the bowl and refrigerate for at least thirty minutes to allow the flavors to meld.
5. Serve the tuna tartare on crostini or crackers and garnish with additional capers and parsley, if desired.

Prep time: 15 minutes (plus 30 minutes of chilling time)

Chapter 6

Dessert

Dark chocolate dipped strawberries with sauce

Ingredients:
- One lb fresh strawberries, washed and dried
- 8 oz dark chocolate, chopped
- 1/4 cup heavy cream
- 1 tbsp unsalted butter
- 1 tsp vanilla extract

Instructions:
1. Line a baking sheet accordingly with parchment paper.
2. In a heatproof bowl, melt the dark chocolate in the microwave or over a double boiler until smooth.
3. Holding a strawberry by the stem, dip it into the melted chocolate, twirling to coat evenly. Place it on the prepared baking sheet well.
4. Repeat with the remaining strawberries. Place the baking sheet in the refrigerator to allow the chocolate to set very well.
5. In a small saucepan, heat the heavy cream and butter over low heat until the butter has melted.

6. Take away from heat and stir in the vanilla extract. Let the sauce cool slightly.
7. Serve the chocolate-dipped strawberries with the sauce on the side for dipping.
8. Enjoy these delicious treats!

Prep time: 30 minutes

Lemon Poppyseed Muffins

Ingredients:
- 2 cups all-purpose flour
- 1/2 cup sugar
- 2 tsp baking powder
- 1/2 tsp baking soda
- 1/4 tsp salt
- Zest of 1 lemon
- 1/4 cup fresh lemon juice
- 1/2 cup plain yogurt
- 1/2 cup unsalted butter, melted
- 2 eggs
- 1 tsp vanilla extract
- 2 tbsp poppy seeds

Instructions:
1. Preheat the oven to 375°F (190°C) and line a muffin tin with paper liners or grease with cooking spray.
2. In a medium bowl, mix together the flour and sugar, baking powder and baking soda, salt and lemon zest.
3. In a separate bowl, mix together the lemon juice, yogurt, melted butter, eggs, and vanilla extract.
4. Pour the wet ingredients into the dry ingredients and stir/mix until just combined. Do not overmix.
5. Gently fold in the poppy seeds.
6. Divide the batter evenly among the muffin cups, filling each about two-thirds full.

7. Bake in the preheated oven for 18-20 minutes, or until a toothpick inserted into the center of a muffin comes out clean.

8. Take away the muffins from the oven and let them cool in the tin for a few minutes or more before transferring to a wire rack to cool completely.

Prep time: 15 minutes
Baking time: 18-20 minutes
Yield: 12 muffins

CONCLUSION

"The Non-Gallbladder Super Diet Cookbook Dishes" is not just a recipe book, it is a comprehensive guide to reclaiming your health and well-being. With its carefully crafted recipes and tailored dietary advice, this cookbook empowers individuals to make informed choices and take control of their digestive health. Whether you are navigating life without a gallbladder or simply seeking to improve your overall well-being, this invaluable resource serves as a roadmap towards a vibrant and nourishing lifestyle. Embrace the power of healing through food and watch as your health and vitality flourish with every delicious dish you create from this transformative cookbook.

www.ingramcontent.com/pod-product-compliance
Lightning Source LLC
Chambersburg PA
CBHW072057230526
45479CB00010B/1120